A NON-LEGAL THRILLER

Focused Ultrasound Foundation . Charlottesville VA

Focused Ultrasound Foundation
1230 Cedars Court, Suite 206
Charlottesville VA 22903

fusfoundation.org

ISBN 978-1-4951-7940-2

Dear Reader

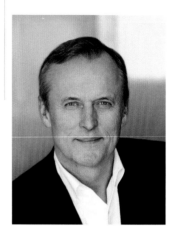

My knowledge of medicine and medical research is quite limited. When I was a student, I drifted away from science and math, preferring instead subjects I considered less demanding. I eventually made it to law school and became a lawyer. After a brief career suing people (never a doctor, though), I stumbled upon fiction and wrote a couple of books. Others followed, and I happily shuttered the law office. Because the books have done well, I have been lucky enough to dabble in philanthropy. Once you get the reputation of being generous, a lot of opportunities present themselves.

Seven years ago, my friend and neighbor, Neal Kassell, gave a PowerPoint presentation on focused ultrasound therapy. Neal is a prominent neurosurgeon who's spent his career drilling through skulls and making repairs to brains. During the PowerPoint, Neal, with great enthusiasm, explained that focused ultrasound therapy could one day alleviate the need for conventional brain surgery. Tumors would be destroyed using beams of ultrasound energy, and afterward the patient would walk out of the operating room and go home. Not only would the treatment be non-invasive, painless, quick, and relatively inexpensive, it could also save the patient's life.

Focused ultrasound therapy is still in its early stages, still experimental, but there is enough research to date to be very optimistic.

The brain is just the starting point. Tumors in the breast, prostate, pancreas, liver, kidneys, and bones could be treated on an out-patient basis. Neal loves to use the example of a man with prostate cancer undergoing focused ultrasound therapy, then driving himself back to the office for a few hours. Later, he goes home to celebrate his wedding anniversary with his wife. They share a champagne toast to growing old together.

This is not science fiction. Around the world, 50,000 men with prostate cancer have been treated with focused ultrasound. Over 22,000 women with uterine fibroids (benign tumors of the uterus) have been treated, thus avoiding hysterectomies and infertility. Clinical trials for tumors of the brain, breast, pancreas and liver, as well as Parkinson's disease, arthritis, and hypertension are inching forward at over 225 research sites around the world.

Though focused ultrasound technology is in its infancy, there is great enthusiasm for its potential to improve the quality of life and decrease the cost of care. This potential, though, remains to be fully demonstrated through additional laboratory research and clinical trials.

But progress is too slow. There are barriers from regulators, insurance companies, even many in the medical field.

I have found no other cause, issue, non-profit, or charity that can potentially save so many lives. One day in the not-too-distant future, you or someone you love will be diagnosed with a tumor. After the shock, you will think of focused ultrasound.

Let's hope it's available.

Chapter 1

The Patient

Meet Paul, a 35-year-old banker with a lovely wife, Karen, and three small children. They enjoy a nice life in the suburbs with lots of friends and the usual activities—backyard cookouts, swim parties, tee-ball, church on Sundays. They are active and enjoy great health. Paul's parents are in their 60s and also very healthy. Paul gets a complete physical once a year, jogs twenty miles a week, plays golf and tennis at a nearby club, and avoids extra pounds. He has an occasional beer, doesn't smoke, and takes no medication.

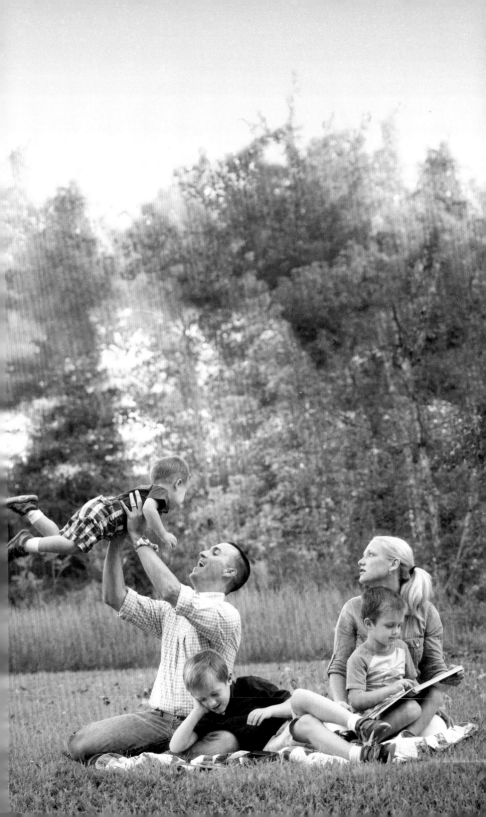

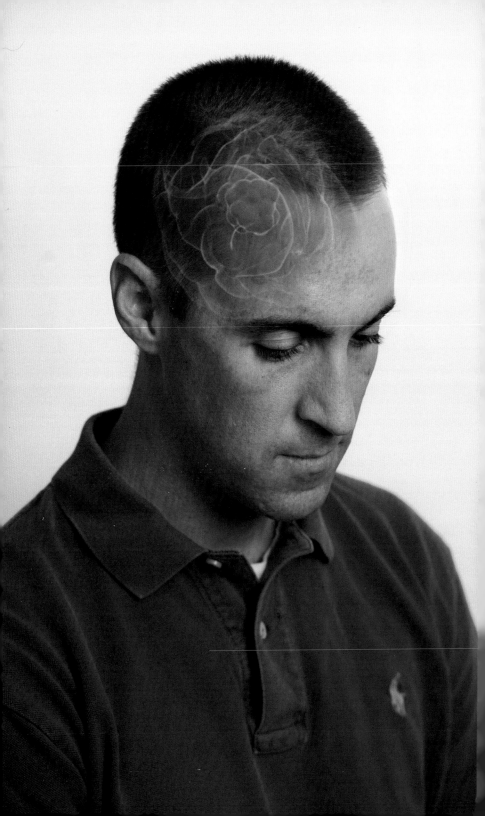

Chapter 2

The Tumor

But Paul has a problem. He has a tumor in the right frontal lobe of his brain, about the size of a hen's egg.

Looking back, the first symptom was a gradual decrease in his ability to concentrate at work. Naturally curious and active, he noticed an uncharacteristic tendency to procrastinate. At times he felt listless and tired. Then the headaches arrived, and with a fury. He blamed them on stress and took lots of ibuprofen. As he drove to work one morning, his vision became so blurred he stopped the car. Karen began to notice mood swings and a loss of patience with the kids. He grew more irritable, both at home and at the office. His boss chastised him for barking at a coworker. He quarreled with Karen over his dour moods and crankiness. She knew something was changing with her husband and urged him to see a doctor. He refused.

On a Wednesday morning, as Paul is in the bathroom shaving, Karen hears a loud thump. She finds him on the floor, shaking in a full-blown grand mal seizure. She calls 911, and as she waits the seizure stops and he gradually awakens. He is confused, disoriented—doesn't recognize Karen and doesn't know where he is. The rescue squad arrives. Paul is loaded into an ambulance and taken to the hospital. In the emergency room, he is still drowsy and confused and complains of weakness on his left side. Upon examination, his left hand is very weak and he has difficulty lifting his left arm and leg. An MR scan reveals the tumor.

He is admitted to the hospital and started on anticonvulsant medication to prevent further seizures, as well as steroids to decrease the swelling in his brain around the tumor. Paul and Karen are not shown the MR scan. A neurosurgeon is consulted.

By Thursday morning, the confusion and disorientation are gone, as is the weakness in his left side. He feels much better, briefly, but things will change. When the neurosurgeon arrives early that morning for the initial consultation, he produces the MR scan (opposite). As they stare at it, Paul and Karen are too stunned to speak. The doctor explains that Paul indeed has a tumor in his brain and it appears to be the type known as a glioma. Surgery is needed to remove as much of it as possible and to obtain tissue to determine the type of tumor.

They talk about the operation. The doctor covers the risks. For complications like death and paralysis, the risks are very small. The most likely complication will be a weakness on the left side. The surgery will take about three hours, and if all goes well, Paul can expect to go home in three days.

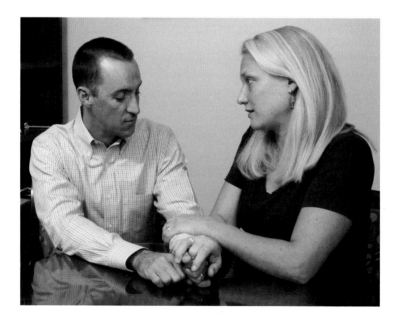

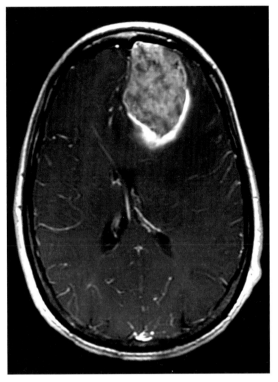
MR scan of Paul's tumor

The neurosurgeon explains that gliomas are graded one through four, with one and two being benign. Three and four are malignant. Grade four, the most catastrophic, is called a glioblastoma. The life expectancy for a grade four diagnosis is short. Regardless of treatment—surgery, chemo, radiation—the average length of survival is about one year. Left untreated but managed with pain medication only, the patient can expect to live several months. About 22,000 Americans are diagnosed each year with glioblastomas; 15,000 die within 12 months. The lucky ones, about one in ten, live for five years.

Based on the MR scan, the neurosurgeon thinks the odds are about 50–50 that the tumor is benign.

He recommends surgery at the earliest convenient time and it is scheduled for the following Monday. After the doctor leaves, Paul and Karen attempt to come to grips with what's happening. Should they get another opinion? It seems senseless when staring at the MR scan. There is no doubt about the tumor. They like their neurosurgeon and a quick search online proves he's one of the best. They are in the finest hospital in the city. Surgery is needed sooner rather than later. There is no time to waste.

Needless to say, the weekend is long and agonizing. Karen gives the bad news to the family but not to their children. She refuses to believe the tumor is malignant and is convinced the surgery will go well.

She spends hours online gathering frightening and depressing information about brain tumors. Ted Kennedy, Susan Hayward, Beau Biden, Lee Atwater, George Gershwin, Lou Rawls, Bobby Van, Pete Rozelle, Wilma Rudolph—they are just a few of those who died from a glioblastoma. On average, they survived a year after being diagnosed.

Opposite

Well-known people who died from a glioblastoma. On average, they survived a year after diagnosis.

top, left to right
Lee Atwater, 40
Wilma Rudolph, 54

middle, left to right
George Gershwin, 38
Edward "Ted" M. Kennedy, 77

bottom, left to right
Joseph Robinette "Beau" Biden, III, 46
Susan Hayward, 57

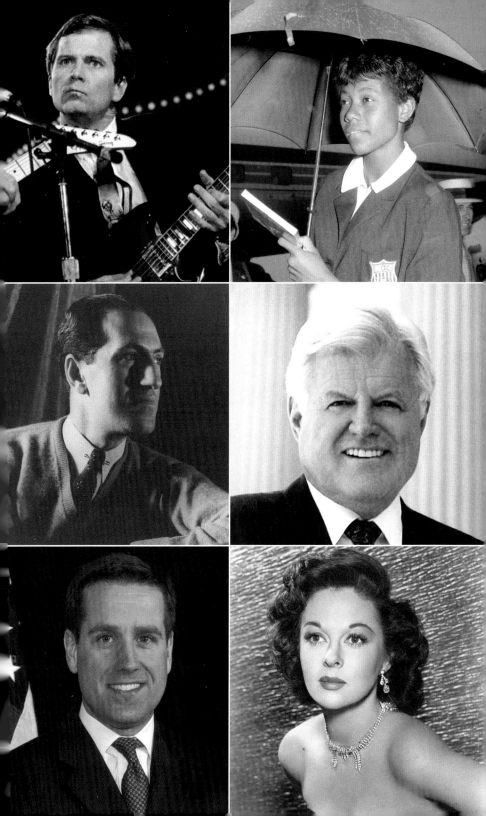

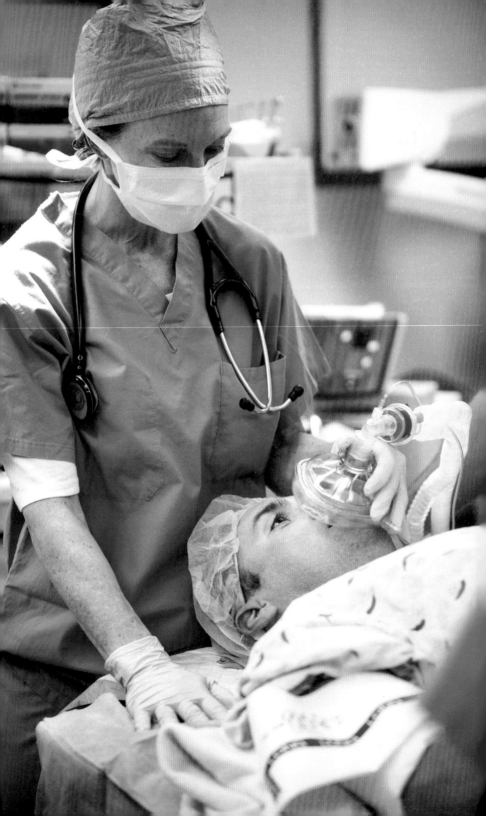

Chapter 3

The Treatment

At 6 a.m. on Monday, Paul and Karen are in his hospital room, wide-awake, fearful but trying to appear brave as they wait for the day to unfold.

At 6:30, Paul is prepped for surgery and two orderlies arrive with a gurney for the short ride to the operating room. Paul hugs his wife, who's overcome with emotion. After he's gone, she is led by a nurse to the waiting room. His parents are already there. The nurse tells them the surgery should be over around noon. As they settle in for a long morning, the room begins to fill with other anxious families.

Paul is rolled into the operating room and put to sleep with general anesthesia.

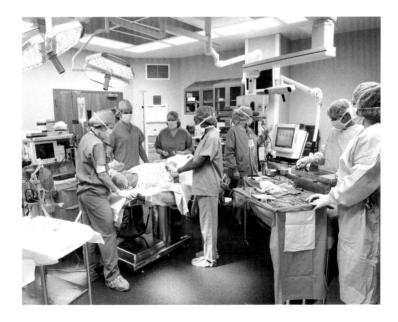

His head is shaved and his skull fixed in a three-prong headrest to immobilize it (fig. 1).

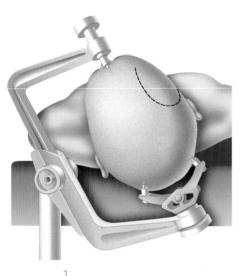

1

A question-mark-shaped incision is made from the midpoint of his forehead just below the hairline to a point in front of his right ear.

Burr holes are made in the skull, and a power saw is used to fashion a bone flap more or less like the top of a cookie jar (fig. 2).

The dura mater—a membrane between the inner table of the skull and the brain—is cut (fig. 3). The surface of the frontal lobe is discolored and distorted because of the tumor.

The tumor is localized with an intraoperative navigation device to minimize damage to the motor cortex—the portion of the brain controlling movement of the left side of the body. Under the magnification of an operating microscope, an incision is made into the brain, and just beneath this the abnormal tissue is identified.

A portion is cut out and sent to the pathology lab for a preliminary diagnosis (fig. 4). The tumor is removed by suction and the bleeding is controlled with coagulation (fig. 5).

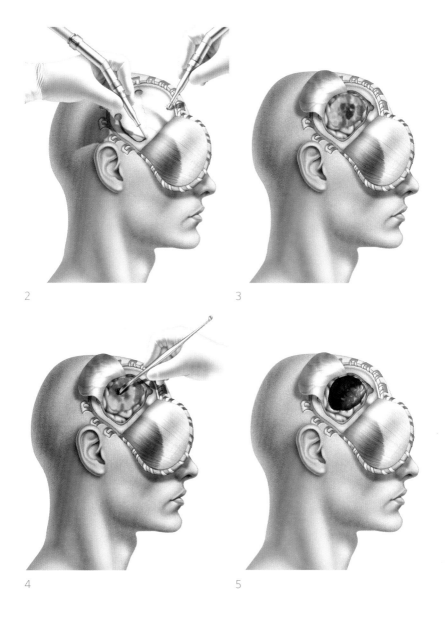

2

3

4

5

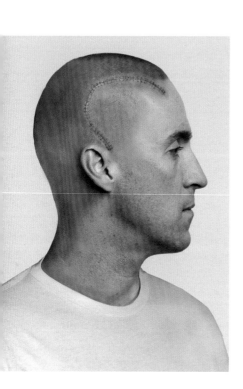

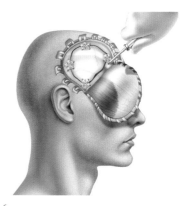

6

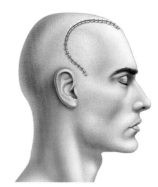

7

The surgeons are able to remove everything that appears abnormal.

They then suture the dura mater, secure the bone flap with screws (fig. 6), and staple the skin flap (fig. 7).

After three hours of surgery, they are confident things went as well as possible. Paul is taken to recovery.

The surgeon goes to the waiting room and meets with Karen and Paul's parents. He reports that everything went as expected: the tumor was removed, there were no complications, and they should be able to see Paul in about an hour. The initial results of the biopsy are not good—it looks like a glioblastoma, but it will take several days for the final report.

Meanwhile, Paul is waking up, and there are problems. He has profound weakness in the left side of his body. He cannot lift his left arm or leg off the bed. He has only a flicker of motion in his fingers. The surgeon immediately orders a CT scan to make sure the weakness is not caused by hemorrhaging or a blood clot in his brain from the surgery. It is not. The CT scan is unremarkable.

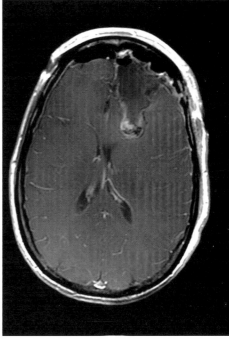

Post-operative MR scan

Early Monday evening, Paul and Karen meet with the neurosurgeon, who has a preliminary pathology report; the final one is a few days away. While the tumor was successfully removed, it is the type of tumor that will likely recur.

The next day another MR scan confirms that there was total removal of all visible tumor, a rare bit of good news (above).

Chemotherapy and radiation will be necessary to slow its regrowth. As for the weakness in Paul's left side, the doctor says it is undoubtedly the result of surgical manipulations and should get better.

By Tuesday morning, the weakness has improved slightly. Paul is able to lift his arm but movements of his fingers are slow and his grip is weak. He is able to stand but can walk only with assistance. Karen stays by his side as the hours drag on. He wants to discuss what's on his mind: death, life insurance, his last

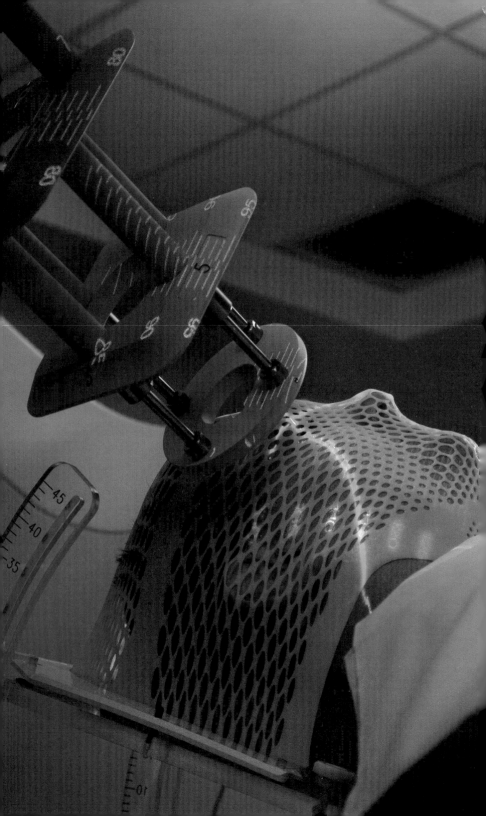

will and testament, their savings, her future, the kids' futures. Karen, though, is simply not ready for this. She doggedly maintains a veneer of optimism. To Paul, it seems more like denial. She tells him that a lot of friends are eager to stop by for a visit, but he says no. He looks awful, feels worse, and wants to see no one, not even his own children.

Early Wednesday morning, one week after his seizure, they meet again with the neurosurgeon. The pathology report confirms their worst fears: glioblastoma, grade four. Although the tumor has been removed, it left behind microscopic portions that extend into the normal brain and cannot be surgically removed. These remnants of the tumor will almost certainly regrow, and must be treated with radiation and chemotherapy. When the tumor returns, there will be the likelihood of more surgery.

With as much professional sympathy as possible, the doctor tells them that, according to statistics, Paul can expect to live 12 to 14 months. Occasionally a patient will live 5 to 10 years, but that's uncommon. He offers his usual, "Hope for a miracle, but plan for the average."

"Plan for the average," Paul repeats after the doctor leaves. Karen pulls the shades and turns off the lights. They sit in the darkness, holding hands, as the monitors beep occasionally. When they speak, they discuss the best way to tell the children.

Thursday morning, the radiation oncologist stops by. He describes radiation therapy and explains that it will be administered five days a week for the next six weeks. Among other side effects, Paul will lose his hair and his face will swell and become disfigured from the steroids he'll be given. Later, the neuro-oncologist stops by and they discuss chemotherapy, which has its own set of unpleasant side effects.

On Friday, Karen brings their children to the hospital to visit. She and Paul have decided to wait a few months before delivering the bad news. They still believe in miracles and are praying a lot. After the kids leave, Paul's parents

Opposite, radiation therapy treatment

visit him. With Karen home with the children, he does not pull punches. He'll be lucky if he's still living a year from now.

Later, alone and in a dark room, Paul opens his laptop and pulls up a calendar for the next 12 months. It's all there, all planned: the school year, their upcoming vacation, the holidays and birthdays, a golfing trip with his friends, several business trips, his parents' 40th anniversary. Would he be able to enjoy any of it? Would he even be alive? "Plan for the average" means he should be able to make it to Christmas. What does a father of three young children do to celebrate his last Christmas?

Paul thinks about the next 12 months and asks himself many questions. There are no answers.

Later that afternoon, he is transferred to a rehabilitation facility to address the weakness in his left side. He cannot raise his left hand to his face, nor can he walk without a cane. Ten days after surgery, he is discharged and taken home. He is instructed to return to the rehab facility three times per week. His left side continues to improve.

Being at home lifts his spirits. Friends arrange meals and there is a steady flow of traffic to the house. He tries to eat but his appetite is gone. Two weeks after surgery, Karen drives him to the office where he's greeted like a hero. He is determined to work at least half a day until he regains his strength, and he assures his colleagues he'll be back. Paul begins radiation therapy Monday through Friday, five days per week.

His hair falls out rapidly from the radiation and, worse, his face begins to swell from the steroids (opposite). The moon face seems to grow each day. He looks terrible. He is constantly fatigued, and his thinking becomes slow and dull from the damage to his brain caused by the radiation.

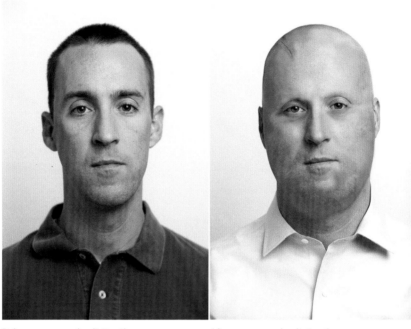

Before surgery and radiation therapy   After surgery and radiation therapy

He gives up on the idea of going to the office. His boss promises to cover for him and keep the paychecks coming. The group medical policy covers 80 percent of the expenses.

His lawyer drafts a new will, not that one is really needed. Paul and Karen own everything jointly; upon his death, it's all hers anyway. She certainly gets the kids. His life insurance policy is for only $250,000. They have about $40,000 in savings. With three children under the age of eight, the future is anything but secure. Karen secretly begins checking out employment opportunities on the internet. Their minister stops by every other day for a devotion and prayer.

Chapter 4

The End

Six months later, the weakness in Paul's left side increases dramatically. He cannot grasp objects with his left hand. He drags his left foot when walking and cannot move around without assistance. He notices he cannot concentrate for more than a few seconds. His short-term memory is shot. An MR scan shows the tumor is back and growing rapidly (below).

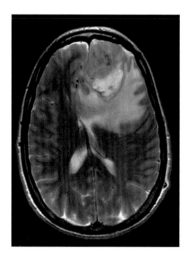

MR showing recurrent tumor

It also reveals damage in his brain compatible with the effects of radiation. His neurosurgeon offers the option of another surgery to remove the recurrent tumor.

Paul and Karen discuss this for several days. A second operation is more likely to damage the brain. There is no certainty that the tumor will not recur again, and again. They are losing hope, and their thoughts of miracles are fading rapidly. Paul could almost throw in the towel, opt for a few final weeks with pain medication, and suffer as little as possible to the end. Karen, though, still believes in luck.

The second operation is similar to the first. The visible portions of the tumor are removed, and Paul's skull is put back together. When he awakens, though, the weakness in his left side is much worse. He is transferred to a rehabilitation center. After three weeks of intense therapy, his condition does not improve. He can no longer stand without assistance, nor walk without a walker. His left hand is essentially useless. He is discharged home,

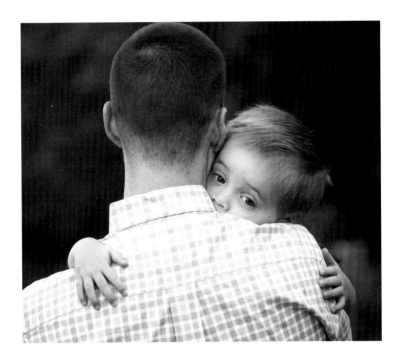

where he arrives in a wheelchair. The chemotherapy has been ineffective and is terminated. Paul takes steroids in an effort to reduce swelling in his brain.

At this point, Paul begins saying goodbye to his family and friends. He bravely accepts the fact that his days are numbered, and he wishes to say farewell on his terms. As bad as he looks, he knows that things will only get worse.

In a heart-wrenching scene, he and Karen finally tell the children that their father is about to leave them.

The steroids are not working and are cut off. He's left with only some powerful narcotics to deaden the horrible headaches, which occur with increasing severity.

Paul prays for a quick and painless end, but this doesn't happen. He slowly deteriorates and becomes increasingly confused and disoriented. He loses almost all consciousness and his ability to move. He is bedridden and requires around-the-clock care for feeding and bathing. Karen sleepwalks through the days and nights, thoroughly drained, but trying gamely to shield his condition from the children as much as possible. Eight months · after his seizure, Paul has completely checked out, but his heart still manages to beat. Karen finally begins praying for a merciful end.

Nine months after the first surgery, he passes away, at the age of 36.

The total cost of his treatment and care is approximately $300,000.

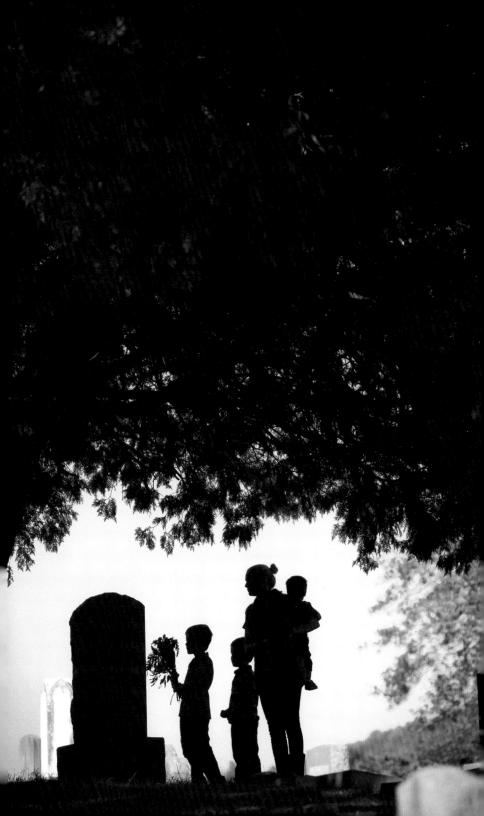

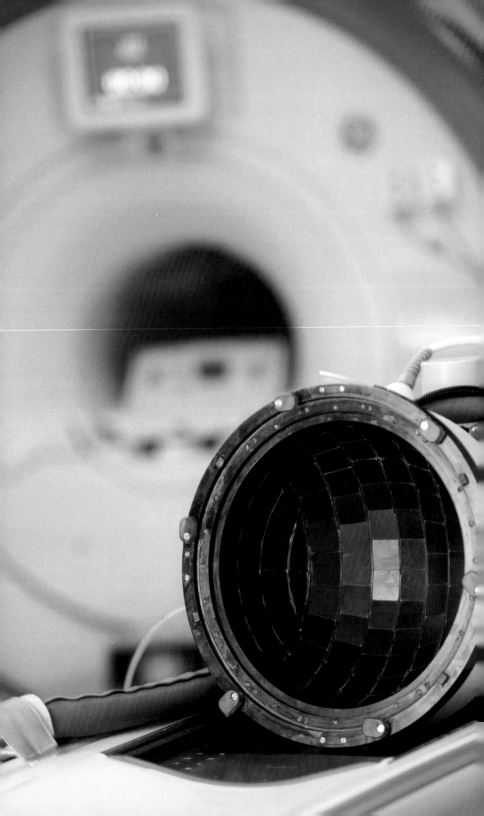

Chapter 5

The Alternative

Paul was born in 1980, ten years too early. Had he been born in 1990 and diagnosed with a brain tumor at the age of 35, in 2025, his story could be rewritten as follows:

That same Wednesday morning, Karen hears a crash in the bathroom, and she finds Paul on the floor in a grand mal seizure. He's taken to the ER and admitted to the hospital. An MR scan is performed with molecular imaging, a more advanced scan than was available ten years earlier.

Based on the scan, the neurosurgeon, with virtual certainty, makes a diagnosis of a glioblastoma and explains the prognosis and the treatment options, including focused ultrasound therapy. The size and location of Paul's tumor make it amenable to treatment with focused ultrasound therapy, which is what the neurosurgeon recommends. He explains that the tumor in all probability cannot be cured and will return, but it can be controlled with repeated treatment, giving Paul more years with a high quality of life.

Opposite, the focused ultrasound brain transducer fits over the head and emits beams of energy that penetrate the skull to target a tumor.

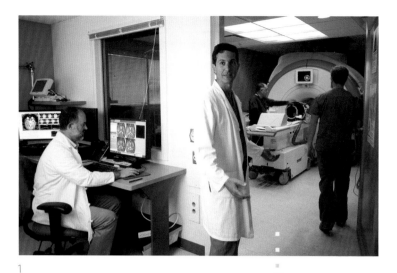

1

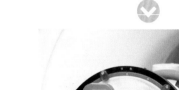
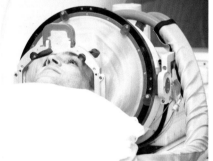

2

Early Friday morning, Paul and Karen walk into the focused ultrasound therapy suite (fig. 1). He changes into a gown, takes a light sedative, and is positioned on his back on a table.

His head is securely fixed in a hemispheric focused ultrasound brain transducer (fig. 2). The transducer is capable of transmitting more than 1,000 intersecting beams of ultrasound energy through the scalp and skull to the tumor with a high degree of accuracy and without damaging the adjacent normal tissue. After the transducer is in place, Paul is inserted into the bore of the MR machine.

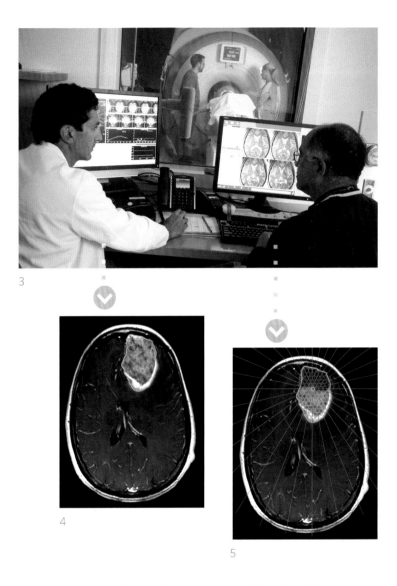

3

4

5

In the adjacent control room, the surgeon manually outlines the tumor, which is to be destroyed by the focused ultrasound beams (fig. 4). Paul is awake and feels no discomfort. Karen stays by his side, holding his hand and chatting with him. The treatment begins. The surgeon is in constant voice contact with Paul and Karen (fig. 3). He uses continuous images from the MR scan to guide the precise point where the ultrasound is focused and to control the delivery of its energy to the target (fig. 5).

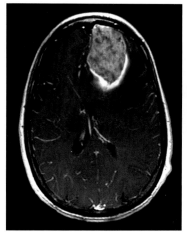
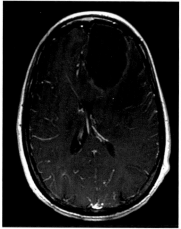

Before focused ultrasound therapy   After focused ultrasound therapy

It takes about an hour to kill all of the tumor that can be seen on the MR. At the completion of the procedure, another MR scan is performed to confirm the entire tumor was treated.

While this is happening, powerful chemotherapy agents enclosed in microscopic nanoparticles are injected intravenously. These circulate with the blood in every tissue and organ in the body, but the chemotherapy drugs are inactive because they are trapped inside the nanoparticles. After eliminating all of the tumor that can be seen on the MR, the surgeon then refocuses the ultrasound to the surrounding brain to activate the nanoparticles, which release their pharmacological payload in the precise area around the tumor where residual microscopic extensions of the tumor have infiltrated. This allows very high concentrations of the drugs to be delivered focally to the brain while minimizing systemic side effects. The remainder of the chemo-laden nanoparticles will be excreted.

Less than two hours after the treatment began, Paul gets off the table and walks to the recovery room for observation. There are no complications, and he is discharged home Friday afternoon. He feels fine. The only aftershock is some residual clumsiness in his left hand from his initial seizure, which is decreasing. On Saturday afternoon, he and Karen and the kids walk down the street for a block party. They have yet to tell their families and friends about the tumor and the treatment. On Sunday, the entire family goes to church.

On Monday, Paul is at the office before 8 a.m., eager to catch up after three days off. He explains to his colleagues that he was in the hospital for "tests," but everything is fine. He looks and feels like himself. The weakness in his left side continues to fade away.

A month after the ultrasound procedure, he undergoes another MR scan. The scan reveals that the ablated tissue is being absorbed harmlessly by Paul's body. The mass is not regrowing due to the efficacy of the focused chemotherapy treatment that targeted the microscopic extensions of the malignant tumor. The deadened tissue continues to shrink.

Three years later, Paul again notices difficulty using his left hand. His left foot occasionally drags. He does not hesitate and calls his doctor immediately. An MR scan is done and reveals that the tumor is back. The following day, as an outpatient, he undergoes another focused ultrasound procedure. The weakness goes away after a month. Four years later, seven years after his initial diagnosis, the tumor is growing again, and the procedure is done for the third time.

Cost to date: approximately $75,000
Savings: about $225,000 and one life prolonged

Chapter 6

The End—Revised Version

The tumor will eventually take Paul's life. However, focused ultrasound therapy could transform a fatal condition into one that is chronic, but manageable. In contrast to the best current treatment circa 2015, the futuristic ultrasound therapy depicted here circa 2025 could potentially be accomplished on an outpatient basis without multiple days of hospitalization; without surgery and its attendant risks of infection and complications like blood clots and brain damage; without the harmful effects of radiation; and with minimal side effects of chemotherapy due to focused drug delivery. The net result could be a dramatic improvement in the quality and longevity of countless lives, and decreased cost of treatment.

How many years will it add? At this time, the answer is uncertain. Clinical trials for brain tumors have just begun, and the patients selected for these trials represent the most desperate of cases. Much more research is needed.

Researchers believe, with caution, that five additional years are realistic. Perhaps ten.

Who wouldn't bargain for ten more years, especially with a high quality of life?

With time, research, and improved technology, neurosurgeons are hopeful that a guy like Paul can live to the age of 45 or even 50, long enough to see his children mature.

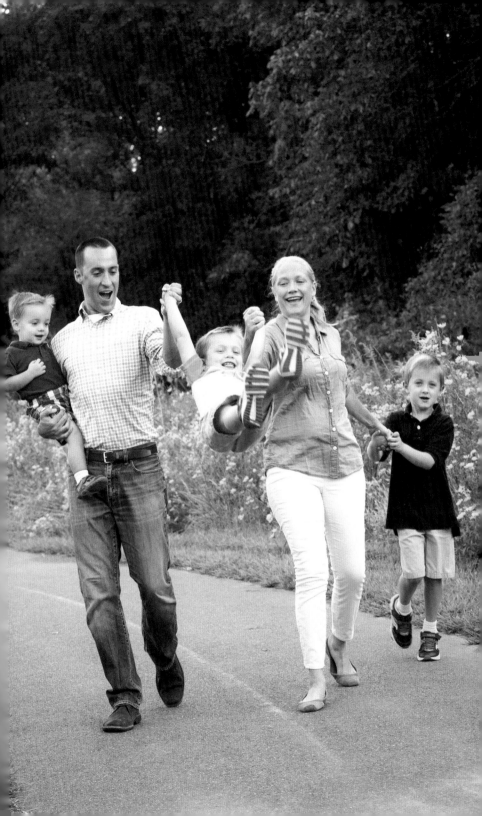

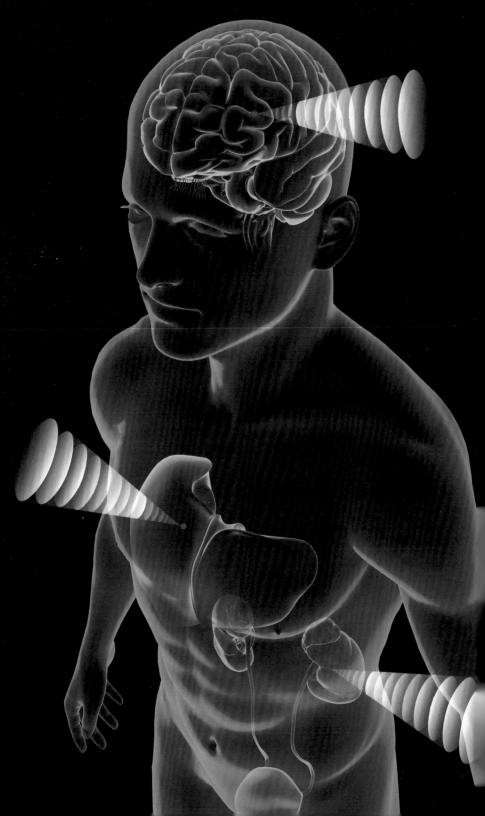

Chapter 7

The Present

Focused ultrasound is a new, revolutionary, groundbreaking, non-invasive therapeutic technology that has the potential to transform the treatment of a variety of serious medical disorders in addition to brain tumors, improve outcomes, and decrease the cost of care. It could become an alternative to, or complement for, traditional surgery, radiation therapy, and drug delivery. Focused ultrasound could result in fewer complications, such as damage to normal tissue, infection, hemorrhage, and pain, as well as shorten recovery times. By providing safer and more effective therapy, it could reduce death, disability, and suffering for millions of people around the world.

Focused ultrasound utilizes intersecting beams of high-frequency sound concentrated accurately and precisely on tissue deep in the body, much as sunlight passing through a magnifying glass can be focused to burn a hole in a leaf.

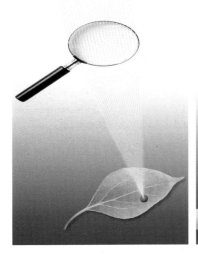
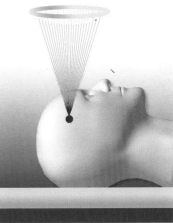

Table 1

Effects at focal point

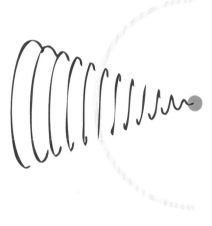

Variety of effects, variety of disorders...

- **Thermal ablation**
  precise heating and destruction of tissue

- **Focal drug delivery**
  delivery of very high concentrations of drugs precisely where they are needed

- **Blood-brain barrier opening**
  temporary access of drugs to reach the brain

- **Immunomodulation**
  stimulation of immune response to allow body to fight cancer

- **Neuromodulation**
  reversible stimulation or inhibition of cells in the brain and nervous system

- **Radiation sensitization**
  sensitizing tumors to effects of radiation allowing use of lower dose to kill cancer cells

- **Stem cell delivery**
  specific "homing" of stem cells to targeted tissue

At the point where the beams converge, the ultrasound energy induces a variety of biological effects while surrounding structures and tissues remain undamaged (table 1).

Magnetic resonance or ultrasound imaging is used to identify, guide, and control the treatment in real time.

In the theoretical example used in this all too common story, focused ultrasound treatment of the malignant brain tumor controlled but did not eradicate it. The alternative treatment provided years of high quality of life to a patient with an ultimately fatal condition. The treatment of brain tumors is not the only area of medicine in which focused ultrasound therapy shows promising results. There are many more applications, including uterine fibroids, prostate cancer, and essential tremor, where focused ultrasound treatment could potentially cure the disease.

Today, focused ultrasound is in various stages of development for treating over 50 diseases and conditions, including hypertension, Alzheimer's and Parkinson's diseases, and tumors of the brain, liver, pancreas, and lung (table 2). But despite the progress so far, much work remains to be done before focused ultrasound can be widely used to treat large numbers of patients.

Unfortunately, it often takes decades for a new therapeutic technology like focused ultrasound to become widely adopted as a mainstream standard of care.

Table 2

Status of progress by disease

	Conceptual Research	Pre-clinical Research	Clinical Trials	Outside US Approval	FDA Approval

Cardiovascular
Disease	Conceptual	Pre-clinical	Clinical Trials	Outside US	FDA
Hypertension	✓	✓			
Atherosclerosis	✓	✓			
Atrial fibrillation	✓	✓			
Peripheral artery disease	✓	✓			
Deep vein thrombosis	✓	✓			
HLHS	✓	✓			
Septal perforation	✓	✓			

Endocrine Disorders
Disease	Conceptual	Pre-clinical	Clinical Trials	Outside US	FDA
Thyroid nodules	✓	✓	✓	✓	
Diabetes	✓	✓			
Obesity	✓	✓			

Miscellaneous
Disease	Conceptual	Pre-clinical	Clinical Trials	Outside US	FDA
Glaucoma	✓	✓	✓		
Hypersplenism	✓	✓	✓		

Musculoskeletal
Disease	Conceptual	Pre-clinical	Clinical Trials	Outside US	FDA
Back & neck pain	✓	✓	✓	✓	
Osteoid osteoma	✓	✓	✓	✓	
Osteoarthritis	✓	✓			
Disc degeneration	✓	✓			
Sacroiliitis	✓	✓			
Spinal cord injury	✓	✓			
Spinal tumors	✓	✓			

Women's Health
Disease	Conceptual	Pre-clinical	Clinical Trials	Outside US	FDA
Uterine fibroids	✓	✓	✓	✓	✓
Breast cancer	✓	✓	✓	✓	
Breast fibroadenoma	✓	✓	✓		
Uterine adenomyosis	✓	✓	✓		
Tubal pregnancy	✓	✓			
Cystic ovary syndrome	✓	✓			
Fetal surgery	✓	✓			

Neurological
Disease	Conceptual	Pre-clinical	Clinical Trials	Outside US	FDA
Essential tremor	✓	✓	✓	✓	
Neuropathic pain	✓	✓	✓		
Parkinson's disease	✓	✓	✓		
Brain tumors	✓	✓	✓		
OCD	✓	✓	✓		
Depression	✓	✓	✓		
Alzheimer's disease	✓	✓			
Epilepsy	✓	✓			
Hydrocephalus	✓	✓			
Stroke	✓	✓			
Traumatic brain injury	✓	✓			
Trigeminal neuralgia	✓	✓			

Oncological
Disease	Conceptual	Pre-clinical	Clinical Trials	Outside US	FDA
Bone metastases	✓	✓	✓	✓	✓
Prostate cancer*	✓	✓	✓	✓	✓
Breast cancer	✓	✓	✓	✓	
Kidney tumors	✓	✓	✓	✓	
Liver tumors	✓	✓	✓	✓	
Pancreatic tumors	✓	✓	✓	✓	
Soft tissue tumors	✓	✓	✓	✓	
Head & neck cancer	✓	✓	✓		
Ovarian cancer	✓	✓			
Colon cancer	✓	✓			
Esophageal cancer	✓	✓			
Lung cancer	✓	✓			

Urological
Disease	Conceptual	Pre-clinical	Clinical Trials	Outside US	FDA
BPH*	✓	✓	✓	✓	✓
Prostate cancer*	✓	✓	✓	✓	✓
Kidney tumors	✓	✓	✓	✓	
Kidney stones	✓	✓	✓		
Acute kidney injury	✓	✓			
Acute tubular necrosis	✓	✓			
Ureterocele	✓	✓			

*The FDA approved two focused ultrasound systems in 2015 that could be used to treat these prostate diseases.

Table 3

Organizations with different agendas

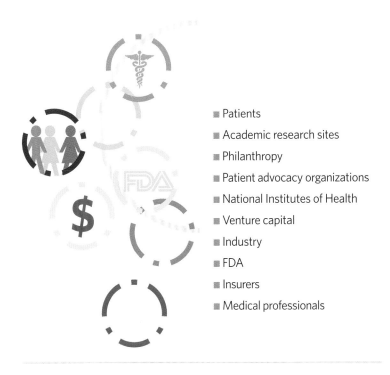

- Patients
- Academic research sites
- Philanthropy
- Patient advocacy organizations
- National Institutes of Health
- Venture capital
- Industry
- FDA
- Insurers
- Medical professionals

Every delay in the availability of focused ultrasound results in unnecessary death, disability, and suffering for countless people.

There are numerous steps in the complicated process of evolution from an idea to laboratory research to widespread patient treatment.

It requires the involvement of a large number of organizations that have different agendas and timelines for decision making (table 3).

Table 4

Obstacles

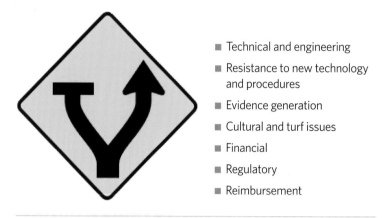

- Technical and engineering
- Resistance to new technology and procedures
- Evidence generation
- Cultural and turf issues
- Financial
- Regulatory
- Reimbursement

Regulatory approvals from the government, reimbursement from insurance companies, and acceptance by physicians are barriers that must first be overcome (table 4).

Research is ongoing in more than 225 academic institutions around the world, including Stanford, University of Virginia, Sunnybrook in Toronto, Royal Marsden in London, and Brigham and Women's. Thirty medical device manufacturers, in partnership with public institutions and patient organizations, are making tremendous progress in understanding and utilizing the mechanisms by which focused ultrasound affects tissue. This knowledge is being converted into laboratory studies and clinical trials which are critical for the ultimate goal—adoption.

The field is growing more rapidly than anticipated, but the amount of work remaining to move this early-stage research into widespread adoption is still great. Additional resources are needed to bridge the gap between research and trials and treating millions of patients with disabling or life-threatening disorders.

Meet three people whose lives have been dramatically improved by focused ultrasound therapy.

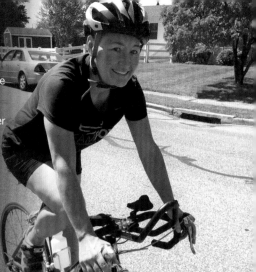

> Six years after her Parkinson's disease diagnosis, Kimberly suffered from involuntary shaking and could no longer ride her bike or enjoy other forms of exercise. She was successfully treated in a focused ultrasound clinical trial at the University of Maryland. She is now back on her bike and says the clock has been turned back on her life.

< Canadian teenager Jack was able to resume his favorite sports after having focused ultrasound treatment for a painful and disabling bone tumor. Before treatment, Jack required heavy doses of pain medications and couldn't sleep through the night. After treatment, his pain went away and he hasn't looked back since.

> Elizabeth suffered from uterine fibroids that made it hard for her to leave the house and work with her interior design clients. Thanks to a focused ultrasound clinical trial, she was able to retain her uterus, eliminate her symptoms, and get back to living.

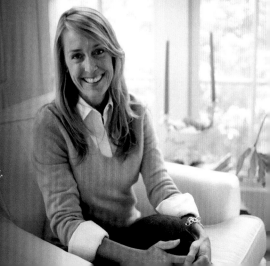

Focused Ultrasound Foundation

In 2006, Dr. Neal Kassell started the Focused Ultrasound Foundation, and headquartered it in his hometown of Charlottesville, Virginia. The Foundation's mission is simple:

> "To accelerate the development and adoption of focused ultrasound."

The Foundation is a unique medical research, education, and advocacy organization whose stated goal is to shorten the time from laboratory research to widespread patient treatment with focused ultrasound. Its principal role is to coordinate the activities of the major players: researchers, doctors, patients, manufacturers, insurers, regulators, and donors. There are now 75 research centers in the U.S. and at least 150 scattered around the world, as well as 30 clinical trials taking place in 11 countries, along with 750 doctors and scientists involved in research and 28 private companies working to perfect the technology. The Foundation is fully engaged with all of these stakeholders.

The Foundation provides resources that are critical to fostering collaboration and generating evidence of the safety and efficacy of focused ultrasound treatments. By doing so, it creates knowledge and allows medical professionals, patients, insurers, and countless other organizations to overcome obstacles, resulting in solutions that help accelerate the development and adoption of focused ultrasound. The metrics of improving the outcome of diagnoses and reducing the cost of care are hard to calculate. But we can estimate that the benefits are immense—particularly when applied to an individual life (table 5).

The Foundation's annual budget is $8 million, 90 percent of which comes from individuals.

Table 5

Time = Lives

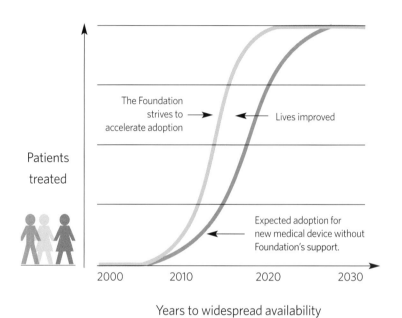

Patients treated

The Foundation strives to accelerate adoption →

← Lives improved

Expected adoption for new medical device without Foundation's support. ←

2000   2010   2020   2030

Years to widespread availability

The Ask

Focused ultrasound is a new, revolutionary, groundbreaking, non-invasive therapeutic technology. In the future, focused ultrasound therapy could be routinely used to treat patients like Paul. Until then, though, millions will suffer and die. "Acceleration" is the operative word, and the Foundation needs your help to speed things along.

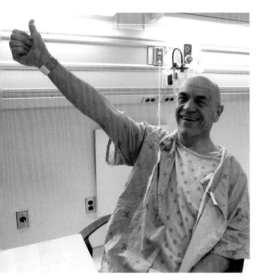

A patient with essential tremor celebrates the return of the use of his right hand after undergoing focused ultrasound treatment.

Visit the Foundation website, www.fusfoundation.org, to:

- Find treatment centers
- Learn about clinical trials
- Sign up to stay in touch
- Support our work
- Share this book

And discover how you could help improve the lives of your friends, loved ones, children—and maybe even your own.

Please remember: Time = Lives.

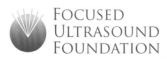

FOCUSED
ULTRASOUND
FOUNDATION

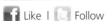

 Like | Follow

Focused Ultrasound Foundation
Board of Directors

Colophon

Designer
Anne Chesnut
Charlottesville VA

Managing editor
Sara Coates Myhre
Charlottesville VA

Copy editor
Margo Browning
Charlottesville VA

Printer
Worth Higgins & Associates, Inc.
Richmond VA

Stock
Endurance Silk text & cover

Type
Galliard, Whitney

Acknowledgements

Focused Ultrasound Foundation would
like to thank Martha Jefferson Hospital
and their Outpatient Care Center for
the generous use of their facilities and
staff in the photography of this book.

Thanks to the following people who
participated in the photography:
Jonathan and Leanna West (Paul and
Karen) and their children Gavin,
Isaac, and Nolan; Shane Allen; Matt
Eames, PhD; Jeff Elias, MD; Sarah Gray;
Thomas E. Huerta; Lee Kassell, MD;
Amber Smith; John Snell, PhD;
Pete Weber; Alexa Witcofsky; and
Kaitlin E. Young.

Photography

Cover, pp. 7, 10, 14, 15, 23, 25, 27, 28,
30, 31, and 35
Stephanie Gross, Charlottesville VA

p. 13 (Lee Atwater)
Office of the President, 21 January 1989

p. 13 (Wilma Rudolph)
Dutch National Archives

p. 13 (George Gershwin),
Library of Congress, Prints and
Photographs Division, Van Vechten
Collection, reproduction number
LC-USZ62-42534 DLC

p. 13 (Edward M. Kennedy)
United States Senate official portrait

p. 13 (Beau Biden)
Official campaign portrait

p. 13 (Susan Hayward)
20th Century Fox publicity photo

p. 46 The Canadian Press/Frank Gunn

MR scans

pp. 11, 19, 24, 31, 32
Max Wintermark, MD,
Stanford University School of Medicine

Illustrations

pp. 16, 17, 18
Anatomical Justice, LLC

pp. 8, 18, 23
Deborah A. Dismuke

pp. 37, 38, 40, 41, 42, 45
Anne Chesnut